I0829541

FROM BMI 30+ TO BMI 18.0 - 24.9: How To Reverse Obesity And Overweight Related Health Conditions.

Dr Robert E. Wright.

All rights reserved. No part of this publication may be reproduced, distributed, or transmitted in any form or by any means, including photocopying, recording, or other electronic or mechanical methods, without the prior written permission of the publisher, except in the case of brief quotations embodied in critical reviews and certain other noncommercial uses permitted by copyright law.

Copyright © Robert E. Wright, 2023.

Table of Contents

Chapter 1: The Concept of BMI

The Body Mass Index (BMI) calculates a person's weight in relation to their height. It is not a precise assessment of a person's total body fat, more of an indicative.

The majority of the time, total body fat and BMI are correlated. This implies that a person's total body fat increases together with their BMI score.

The WHO classifies adults with BMIs of 25 to 29.9 as overweight, adults with BMIs of 30 or higher as obese, adults with BMIs below 18.5 as underweight, and adults with BMIs of 18.5 to 24.9 as healthy weight.

Computation of BMI

BMI is determined for an individual using a mathematical formula. BMI can also be calculated using tables where one can compare weight in pounds to height in inches. BMI calculations can also be done easily with the use of online calculators.

BMI is calculated as follows: (Weight in kilos) / (Height in meters squared)

$$BMI = Weight\ (kg) / Height\ (m)^2$$

A BMI that ranges between 18.5 to 24.9 is considered to be normal. This shows that the person's weight is within the acceptable range for his or her height. An individual is classified as underweight, normal, overweight, or obese using a BMI chart.

Body Mass Index (BMI)	Weight Status
Below 18.5	Underweight
18.5 to 24.9	Normal
25.0 to 29.9	Overweight

30.0 and above	Obes

Classification	BMI Range - kg/m²
Severe Thinness	< 16
Moderate Thinness	16 - 17
Mild Thinness	17 - 18.5
Normal	18.5 - 25
Overweight	25 - 30
Obese I	30 - 35
Obese II	35 - 40
Obese III	> 40

BMI table for children and teens, age 2-20

The BMI classification is advised for kids and teenagers between the ages of 2 and 20, according to the Centers for Disease Control and Prevention (CDC).

Category	Percentile Range
Underweight	< 5%
Healthy Weight	5 - 85%
At Risk of Overweight	85 - 95%
Overweight	> 95%

BMI's clinical relevance

For many people, BMI serves as an indicator of total body fat. As a result, it is regarded as a health risk indicator.

Healthcare workers test for overweight and obese people using BMI. The BMI is used to evaluate a person's risk for obesity and overweight-related health problems.

However, one of the instruments used to determine health risks is BMI. When determining health risks, other factors are also taken into account, including blood pressure, cholesterol, blood sugar, family history of heart disease, age, gender, waist circumference, amount of physical activity, menopause status, smoking status, etc.

Does BMI apply to everyone?

BMI is a reliable indicator of obesity for the majority of people. However, BMI is unable to offer accurate data on body composition, such as the amount of muscle, bone, fat, and other components.

BMI can be a more reliable indicator of body fat in certain people than in others. For instance, exceptionally strong people may be classified as "overweight" even when they are very healthy and athletic. These people may have the same BMI as an overweight person despite having an extremely low body fat percentage.

In a similar vein, an aged and feeble person with minimal muscle mass and a high body fat percentage may fall into the normal weight bracket.

BMI must be carefully evaluated and understood when utilized for growing children and teenagers, people with large or petite frames, pregnant women, and people with a lot of muscle mass

.

Important information

- Since 1975, the global rate of obesity has nearly tripled.

- Over 1.9 billion persons aged 18 and older were overweight in 2016.

- Over 650 million of these people were obese.

- In 2016, 13% of people 18 and older were obese and 39% were overweight.

- The majority of people on earth reside in nations where being overweight or obese kills more people than being underweight.

- In 2020, there were 39 million under-fives who were overweight or obese.

- In 2016, there were approximately 340
  million overweight or obese kids and
  teenagers between the ages of 5 and 19.

- The predicted number of overweight and
  obese people in Nigeria aged 15 or older
  in 2020 was 12 million and 21 million,
  respectively.

- An estimated 2.8 million people each year
  worldwide pass away from obesity-related
  problems.

- Obesity can be avoided.

What are overweight and obesity?

The definitions of overweight and obesity
include abnormal or excessive fat accumulation
that could harm one's health.

In the United States, obesity and overweight are prevalent conditions that are characterized by an increase in the size and number of fat cells in the body. Numerous variables, such as habits including eating habits, insufficient sleep or physical exercise, some medications, genetics, and family history all contribute to being overweight or obese. Obesity is a chronic health condition that increases the risk of heart disease, the top killer in the US, and is connected to several other conditions, such as type 2 diabetes and cancer.

In the United States, over 3 out of 4 persons who are 20 or older are either overweight or obese. Obesity affects around 1 in 5 kids and teens between the ages of 2 and 19. For people of all ages, being overweight or obese can result in major health problems.

Your risk of being overweight and obese can be increased by unhealthy lifestyle choices like not getting enough exercise and consuming foods and drinks that are high in calories but poor in nutrients. When taking medication for a different medical problem, such as diabetes, depression, or high blood pressure, some patients discover that their weight increases.

Following a heart-healthy diet lower in calories and dangerous saturated fats and boosting physical exercise are two lifestyle adjustments that can help people lose weight. Additionally, medications and other weight-loss procedures have received FDA approval. A therapy option that is not always available is surgery.

What contributes to overweight and obesity?

Obesity and overweight are primarily caused by an imbalance in energy between calories consumed and calories burned. Around the world, there have been

- a rise in the consumption of foods with lots of sugar and fat that are high in energy;

- a rise in physical inactivity brought on by the sedentary nature of many jobs, shifting transit options, and growing urbanization.

- A lack of supportive policies in areas like health, agriculture, transportation, urban planning, environment, food processing, distribution, marketing, and education often leads to environmental and societal changes that affect dietary and physical activity patterns.

Obesity and Overweight Health Risks

Obesity and being overweight may increase your risk for specific health issues as well as be related to specific emotional and social issues.

Which health hazards are associated with being overweight or obese?

1. Diabetes Type 2

When blood glucose, also known as blood sugar,
is too high, type 2 diabetes develops. Eight out
of ten individuals with type 2 diabetes are obese
or overweight.8 High blood sugar levels
eventually cause issues like heart disease, stroke,
renal disease, vision problems, nerve damage,
and other medical issues.

Losing 5 to 7 percent of your body weight and
engaging in regular physical activity, if you are
at risk for type 2 diabetes, may help you delay or
avoid the start of the disease.

2. Elevated Blood Pressure

Blood rushes through your blood vessels with
more power than usual when you have high
blood pressure, commonly known as
hypertension. Your risk of heart attack, stroke,
kidney illness, and mortality can all be increased
by high blood pressure, which can also strain
your heart and harm your blood vessels.

3. Heart Disease

The phrase "heart disease" is used to indicate many conditions that could harm your heart. Heart illness increases your risk of experiencing a heart attack, heart failure, sudden cardiac death, angina, or an irregular heart rhythm. Your risk of heart disease may increase if you have high blood pressure, abnormal blood fat levels, or high blood glucose levels. Triglycerides, HDL cholesterol, and LDL cholesterol are all examples of blood fats, commonly referred to as blood lipids.

Your risk factors for developing heart disease may be lowered by losing 5 to 10 percent of your body weight. This could include shedding as little as 10 pounds if you weigh 200 pounds. Blood flow, cholesterol, and blood pressure may all improve with weight loss.

4. Stroke

A blockage or blood vessel break in your brain or neck can result in a stroke, which is a disease when your brain's blood supply is abruptly cut off. Following a stroke, your ability to speak and move some body parts may be lost. Stroke incidence is most commonly caused by high blood pressure.

5. Sleep Apnea

A common disorder called sleep apnea causes irregular breathing while you are asleep. There may be brief instances when you completely cease breathing. Your chance of developing other health issues, such as type 2 diabetes and heart disease, may increase if sleep apnea is left untreated.

6. Metabolic Syndrome

A collection of illnesses known as metabolic syndrome increase your chances of developing diabetes, heart disease, and stroke. These circumstances are

- blood pressure is high.

- high amounts of blood sugar

- excessive amounts of triglycerides in your blood

- your blood has low levels of HDL cholesterol, the "good" cholesterol

- you have too much belly fat

7. Fatty Liver Diseases

Fat builds up in the liver in illnesses known as fatty liver diseases. Nonalcoholic steatohepatitis (**NASH**) and nonalcoholic fatty liver disease (**NAFLD**) are two examples of fatty liver diseases. Cirrhosis, serious liver damage, and even liver failure can result from fatty liver conditions.

8. Osteoarthritis

Osteoarthritis is a chronic health condition that affects many people and results in pain, swelling, and restricted joint motion. Being obese or overweight puts additional strain on your joints and cartilage, which increases your risk of developing osteoarthritis.

9. Gout

Your body may develop needle-like crystals from accumulated uric acid, which would irritate your big toe, ankle, or knee joints. The chance of a flare increases with weight and could potentially be related to insulin resistance. A weight-loss program is a component of controlling gout in obese persons. A heart-healthy diet and regular exercise may help you lose weight and reduce your uric acid levels.

10. Gallbladder Diseases

Obesity and overweight may increase your chance of developing gallbladder conditions like cholecystitis and gallstones. Gallstones are caused by imbalances in the bile's constituent chemicals. If bile contains too much cholesterol, gallstones may develop.

11. Some Cancers

A group of connected disorders make up cancer. All cancers cause a portion of the body's cells to start dividing uncontrollably and spread to neighboring regions. Obesity and overweight may increase your risk of getting some types of cancer.

12. Kidney Disease

Your kidneys are harmed and unable to properly filter blood if you have renal disease. The most frequent causes of kidney disease, diabetes and high blood pressure, are made more likely by obesity. Obesity itself may increase kidney disease and hasten its progression, even if you don't have diabetes or high blood pressure.

13. Obstetrical Issues

Obesity and overweight increase the likelihood of pregnancy-related health issues. Overweight or obese pregnant women may have a higher risk of

- getting pregnant-related diabetes

- experiencing preeclampsia, high blood pressure during pregnancy that, if unchecked, can have serious health effects on both the mother and the unborn child.

- requiring a cesarean surgery (C-section) and, as a result, recovering after childbirth more slowly

What social and mental issues are related to being overweight or obese?

Obesity and overweight are linked to mental health issues including depression. People who struggle with being overweight or obese may also encounter prejudice and stigma related to their weight from others, especially medical professionals. This can exacerbate mental health issues by causing feelings of rejection, shame, or guilt.

Chapter 3: Management of Overweight And Obesity

Losing weight through healthy eating, increasing physical activity, and making other modifications to your regular routines are common therapies for overweight and obesity. Some persons may benefit from weight-management programs in terms of weight loss or preventing weight gain. Some obese persons are unable to maintain their weight loss or drop enough weight to enhance their health. In certain circumstances, a physician might think about incorporating other therapies, such as weight-loss drugs, gadgets, or bariatric surgery.

Five to ten percent of your body weight should be lost over the first six months of treatment, according to experts. [10] This could include shedding as little as 10 pounds if you weigh 200 pounds. 5% to 10% of your weight may be lost by

- reduce your risk of becoming overweight or obese-related health issues

- increase the effectiveness of treatments for obesity-related health issues like high cholesterol and blood pressure.

- healthy eating habits and regular exercise

The first step in attempting to manage overweight and obesity is frequently adopting a healthy eating regimen that contains fewer calories.

People with obesity or excess weight should start a regular exercise regimen at the same time they start a healthy food plan. You might burn more calories if you're active. Your ability to maintain a healthy weight may be aided by regular exercise.

The key to losing and keeping off weight is to change your eating habits. You must consume fewer calories overall and burn more calories than you consume to lose weight. For many people, maintaining this for a longer period might be difficult. New research suggests that following an eating plan consistently may be more crucial for weight loss and maintenance than the sort of food plan you choose.

Adhere to a healthy eating regimen

Every meal and drink option you make counts. Your age, weight, metabolism, food preferences, access to food, culture, and customs, as well as your gender and the decisions you have made in the past, all influence your journey toward a healthy diet. A nutritious diet includes

- a range of fresh produce, whole grains like brown rice, oats, whole-wheat bread, and fruits.

- dairy items including milk, yogurt, and cheese that are fat-free or low-fat, as well as comparable goods like soy beverages

- shellfish, lean meats and poultry, eggs, legumes (beans and peas), almonds, seeds, and soy products are just a few examples of the many protein-rich foods.

- oils, including those found in almonds, avocados, olives, and canola

A nutritious diet program also includes

- ingesting less salt (sodium), processed carbs, and added sugars in food and drink

- limiting serving sizes

- limiting foods high in trans and saturated fats, such as fried and sweet foods.

Engage in regular exercise

Exercise regularly can:

- assist you in losing extra weight

Enhance your physical fitness

several heart disease risk factors, such as "bad" LDL cholesterol levels, should be reduced, while "good" HDL cholesterol levels should be elevated and excessive blood pressure should be controlled.

Reduce stress to enhance your mental well-being.

Reduce your likelihood of developing other diseases like type 2 diabetes, depression, and cancer

Before beginning a new workout regimen, consult your healthcare professional. Talk about the appropriate levels and types of physical activity for you. Physical activity, even in little doses, benefits your health.

Your heart and lungs will benefit most from aerobic activity. Exercise that causes your heart to beat more quickly and causes you to breathe in more oxygen than normal includes brisk walking, jogging, biking, and swimming.

You gain more advantages the more active you are.

Throughout the week, engage in aerobic exercise for at least a few minutes at a time.

Adults should stand up more frequently and sit less. A little exercise is preferable to none.

Adapting your behavior

Although it is challenging to alter your eating and exercise routines and lifestyle, you might be able to reduce your weight and improve your health with a plan, some work, regular support, and patience. The following advice could assist you in coming up with long-term strategies for weight loss, regular exercise, and health improvement.

- Be ready for setbacks; they are expected. Try to refocus after a setback, such as overindulging at a family or work party, and concentrate on returning to your healthy eating plan as soon as you can. Try to limit your eating to times when you are seated at a kitchen or dining room table. Avoid locations where snacks might be offered at work. Use online tools that help you keep track of the meals you eat, your physical activity, and your weight, such as the Body Weight Planner, to monitor your progress. These resources might support your persistence and motivation.

- Set objectives. Setting clear objectives can assist you in staying on course. Instead of aiming to "be more active," decide to walk for 15 to 30 minutes each Monday and Friday before work or at lunch. If you don't go for a stroll on Monday, go for one on Tuesday.

- Seek assistance. Consult with your loved ones, close friends, or medical professionals for advice or support. You can contact support by phone, email, text message, or in person. Another option is to join a support group. You can improve your lifestyle with the assistance of specially trained health professionals.

Programs to manage one's weight

A systematic regimen for weight management helps some people. In a weight-management program, qualified weight-management specialists will create an extensive strategy just for you and assist you in following it. Plans include techniques to assist you to alter your habits and maintain them, as well as a lower-calorie diet, more physical activity, and other measures. You can have individual or group sessions with the specialists in person (on-site). To support your plan, the experts may frequently contact you by phone or online. You may monitor how well you are adhering to your plan using gadgets like smartphones, pedometers, and accelerometers.

Online weight-management programs or commercial weight-loss programs may also be helpful for certain people.

What qualities ought a weight-loss program have?

You must concentrate on your general health and lifestyle choices, not just what you eat if you want to achieve and maintain a healthy weight over the long term. Successful weight-loss programs should encourage healthy habits that can be practiced every day, help you lose weight safely, and keep it off.

Programs for weight loss that are secure and effective need to

behavioral therapy, also known as lifestyle counseling, can help you learn how to create and maintain better eating and exercise routines, such as by keeping food and activity logs or journals.

information on how much sleep is necessary, how to deal with stress, and the advantages and disadvantages of weight-loss medications.

continuous monitoring, support, and feedback throughout the program, whether in person, over the phone, online, or via a combination of these methods.

Weight loss goals should be modest and consistent, averaging 1 to 2 pounds per week (although weight loss may be quicker at the beginning of a program).

a strategy for maintaining weight loss that includes goal-setting, self-evaluations keeping a food journal, and help from counselors.

The most effective weight-loss programs offer behavioral treatment for at least 14 sessions spread over at least six months, and they are run by qualified staff.

Experts advise a starting weight loss goal of 5 to 10% of your starting weight within 6 months for persons who are overweight or obese.
2 If you started at 200 pounds, losing 10 pounds (5 percent) to 20 pounds (10 percent) in six months would result in a loss of that much weight.

Although altering your lifestyle is difficult, you may be able to keep off the weight reduction by establishing good habits that you stick with.

Avoidance of weight loss programs

Avoid diet plans that promise to do any of the following:

- Get in shape without dieting or exercising!

- Eat as many of your favorite meals as you want and still lose weight!

- 30 pounds to lose in 30 days!

- Lose weight in your body's specific trouble spots!

Other cautionary indicators include

- Footnotes, asterisks, and very small types can all make it simple to overlook crucial information.

- Photos of the before and after that appear to be fake

- individual recommendations that might be made up

Weight loss drugs

Your doctor may prescribe medications to treat overweight and obesity if healthy eating and exercise routines are insufficient to address these conditions.

While taking weight-loss medications, you should aim to maintain your healthy eating routine and keep up your normal physical activity.

You could come across advertisements for dietary supplements and herbal therapies that promise to make you lose weight. However, many of these assertions are untrue. Even some of these supplements' severe adverse effects are possible. Before using any over-the-counter herbal medicines or nutritional supplements to aid in weight loss, see your doctor.

Chapter 4: Healthy Meal Plan For Weight Loss

How to Pick a Weight-Loss Program?

You may grow fatigued when attempting to select from the hundreds of weight loss regimens accessible, regardless of whether you need to shed only a few extra kilograms or up to 20 or 60 kilograms. There are many diets for losing weight that calls for consuming particular foods, specific drink concoctions, or weight reduction supplements. Which one, though, is best for you? Utilize these suggestions to pick a weight loss plan that complements your daily schedule and way of life.

What Style Do You Have?

Your style should be reflected in a diet plan for weight loss. It's possible that what works for one individual won't work for you. You should think about your daily schedule, your preferred food groups, and your body's nutritional requirements. Do you like desserts? Do you like to eat meat? Several diets let you to consume moderate amounts of meat and sugar. Think about how many meals you can consume as well. Do you typically eat three large meals per day, or are your meals smaller and more often spaced out? Before beginning a weight loss program, ask yourself these questions to help you identify an easy-to-follow diet that will help you attain your objectives.

Research the Risks

Regarding weight reduction and your health, certain diets are riskier than others. For example, rapid weight loss may be detrimental to the body, particularly if it is sustained for an extended length of time. Taking diet medicines without first contacting a doctor might also be risky. If you have specific medical conditions, some diets can be detrimental to your health. For instance, if you already have cardiac or stomach issues, a diet high in meat might not be the greatest choice. You should see your doctor before beginning a weight loss program if you have any major health issues or are using prescription medication.

Types of Diets for Losing Weight

There are numerous weight loss programs, but they are all unique. Before beginning your weight loss journey, it's a good idea to research the various sorts of plans. Discover the diet for weight loss that is right for you. Think about how each will impact your physical well-being and how each strategy will fit into your schedule or habit. Let's look at the different diet plans that are offered and what is necessary for each.

How to loose weight quickly?

Certain quick diets can help you lose 2–6kg in no time, even if fast weight loss is not advised for the long term. There are several of them, such as the low-carb diet, three- to five-day meal replacement shakes, water or juice fasts, and

alternate fruit/vegetable diets where you
consume only fruits one day and just vegetables
the next. These diets are excellent for a
temporary cure, but they are exceedingly
difficult (and perhaps unhealthy) to keep up over
the long haul.

Low-calorie diets for weight loss

You can limit your daily calorie intake to lose
weight by following one of the several
low-calorie diets available. You can keep an eye
on your calories in a variety of methods. You can
examine food labels and calculate how many
calories are in each meal. To find out how many
calories are in specific meals or dishes that don't
have labels, you can alternatively utilize a
calorie guide. Weight Watchers offers a simple
point counter that determines points based on the
number of calories, grams of fiber, and grams of
fat in meals.

Fixed - menu diet

You will be given a list of all the things you are allowed to eat when following a fixed-menu diet plan. The meal plans are created specifically for you depending on your preferences and requirements. As you shed pounds, this kind of diet can make life easier for you, but bear in mind that you'll eventually have to start organizing your meals once more. So once you've started to lose weight, it's a good idea to understand how to plan your meals. This will assist you in maintaining your weight loss when the fixed-menu diet is over.

What Style Do You Have?

You will schedule meals on an exchange food diet with a predetermined amount of servings from various food groups. Calorie intake determines the foods, and you can choose from a variety of foods that have the same number of calories at each meal. This diet is excellent if you've just finished a set menu diet because it gives you the freedom to choose your meals every day.

A diet low in fat

The low-fat diet is another sort of eating plan that calls for cutting back on fat consumption. This doesn't mean eliminating all fats from your diet; rather, it only means keeping your intake of fats (particularly saturated fats) and oils within the range recommended by the food pyramid. About 30% of the calories consumed should be fat. Saturated fat reduction encourages healthy weight loss and lowers cholesterol to support heart health. Numerous meals with the claim of being "low fat" are highly rich in sugar. For healthy weight loss, look for foods that are low in sugar and fat. Limit your intake of fast food, or choose salads or grilled items from the menu instead. Fast food that is fried often contains a lot of fat.

Losing Weight by Reducing Portion Size

There are also diets for losing weight where you can essentially eat everything you want but the portions are decreased. You eat only a few bites at a time and essentially listen to your stomach. You eat gently till you're satiated but not overstuffed when your stomach is empty. You only consume food when you are truly hungry. This kind of diet allows you to eat everything you want, but it places restrictions on how much you can consume. The idea is that if you eat fewer calories and less food overall at each meal, regardless of what you eat, you will consume less fat and calories overall.

Pre-packaged meals and mixes are also available to aid with weight loss. Any diet can be successful as long as you follow the instructions, add exercise or activity, and drink enough water. Find a diet that works for you by researching each type. If you have a medical condition or are on medication, consult your doctor before beginning a new diet. You can quickly look for diet programs online and obtain a ton of free weight reduction advice to assist you in creating a strategy.

The 9 Healthiest Diets You Can Follow

Many diets have advantages besides just helping you lose weight. The best weight-loss plans enhance general health as well. The hardest part is figuring out which will work for you.

Diets aren't only about losing weight. While altering your food can be one of the most effective ways to lose weight, it can also serve as a springboard for bettering your routines, paying more attention to your health, and living an active lifestyle.

But it could be challenging to begin given the overwhelming quantity of diet programs that are available. For certain people, various diets will be more effective, lasting, and suitable.

While some diets recommend limiting your consumption of calories and either fat or carbohydrates, others focus on reducing your hunger. Some people prioritize changing their eating habits and lifestyles above restricting particular items.

Additionally, several have health advantages beyond weight loss.

Here are the top 9 diets to help you get healthier overall.

1. The Mediterranean diet

The Mediterranean diet has long been regarded as the ideal one in terms of health, longevity, disease prevention, and nutrition. This is based on its sustainable nature and benefits to nutrition.

How it works

The Mediterranean diet is based on foods that have historically been consumed in places like Italy and Greece. It is abundant in

- fruits and veggies,
- whole grains
- olive oil
- lentils
- fish
- nuts

Red meat consumption should be restricted, while foods like chicken, eggs, and dairy products should be consumed in moderation.

The Mediterranean diet also restricts:

- refined foods
- trans fat
- added sugar,
- processed meats, and
- other highly processed foods

Health advantages

This diet's focus on minimally processed foods and plants has been linked to a lower risk of developing a number of chronic diseases as well as a longer life span. Additionally, studies demonstrate that the Mediterranean diet protects against several malignancies.

Numerous studies show that the diet's plant-based, high unsaturated fat nutritional pattern can help with weight loss, despite the fact that it was created to reduce the risk of heart disease.

After a year, the Mediterranean diet produced greater weight loss than a low-fat diet, according to a systematic review that looked at five distinct research. It generated weight loss effects that were comparable to those of a low-carb diet.

In one 12-month trial of more than 500 adults, increased adherence to a Mediterranean diet was linked to a doubled chance of weight loss maintenance.

Additionally, the Mediterranean diet promotes consuming a lot of foods high in antioxidants, which may help fight oxidative stress and inflammation by scavenging free radicals.

Other advantages

The Mediterranean diet is linked to a lower risk of mental diseases, such as depression and cognitive loss, according to recent studies.

A diet that is more sustainable for the environment is also linked to eating less meat.

Downsides

Since dairy products are not heavily emphasized in the Mediterranean diet, it's crucial to make sure your diet has enough calcium and vitamin D.

Summary

Eating a lot of fruits, vegetables, seafood, and healthy fats is emphasized in the Mediterranean diet, while avoiding refined and highly processed foods.

Despite not being a diet for weight loss, research have shown that it can aid in both weight loss and general health.

2. The DASH diet

DASH, or **dietary approaches to stop hypertension**, is an eating strategy created to assist in the treatment or prevention of high blood pressure, also referred to as hypertension.

Eat plenty of fruits, veggies, nutritious grains, and lean meats, it urges. Red meat, salt, added sugars, and fat are all in moderation.

Despite not being a weight loss diet, many people who follow the DASH diet claim to have lost weight.

What it does

The DASH diet suggests particular portions of various food groups. Your daily calorie intake determines how many portions you should consume.

For illustration, a typical DASH dieter would consume roughly:

- five veggie servings
- five fruit servings
- 7 servings of whole grains and other nutritious carbohydrates
- two servings of dairy products with minimal fat
- two servings of lean meats or less

Additionally, eating nuts and seeds two to three times a week is advised.

Health advantages

It has been demonstrated that the DASH diet lowers blood pressure and several heart disease risk factors. It might also aid in reducing your risk of developing colorectal and breast cancer.

According to studies, the DASH diet can also aid in weight loss. For instance, a review of 13 research revealed that those following the DASH diet lost more weight over 8–24 weeks than those following a control diet.

Another 12-week trial of obese people found that while maintaining muscle strength, the DASH diet helped study participants reduce their overall body weight, body fat percentage, and absolute fat mass.

Other advantages

The DASH diet may assist with treating depressive symptoms in addition to weight loss.

Even moderate DASH diet adherence was linked to a lower incidence of depression, according to a comparative study conducted over an eight-year period.

Downsides

While there is conflicting research about salt intake and blood pressure, the DASH diet may help people with hypertension lose weight and drop their blood pressure.

A low-sodium diet isn't the best option for everyone because eating too little salt has been associated with increased insulin resistance.

For people with hypertension or other medical disorders that benefit or necessitate sodium restriction, a low-sodium diet like the DASH diet is more suitable.

To fully comprehend how a low salt diet can influence insulin resistance in people without hypertension, more study is required in this area.

Summary

A low-sodium diet that has been demonstrated to help people lose weight is the DASH diet.

Additionally, studies have connected it to improved heart health and lower risks of developing other chronic conditions.

3. Plant-based and flexitarian diets

The most well-known plant-based diets, which forgo animal products for ethical, environmental, and health grounds, are vegetarianism and veganism.

However, there are also more adaptable plant-based diets, including the flexitarian diet. This is a plant-based diet that permits occasional use of animal products.

What it does

Typical vegetarian diets forbid all forms of meat but permit dairy items. Vegan diets typically forbid the consumption of any animal products, including dairy, butter, and occasionally other byproducts like honey.

The flexitarian eating plan is regarded as more of a lifestyle than a diet because it lacks precise guidelines or recommendations regarding calories and macronutrients. Its tenets consist of:

- ingesting largely fruits, vegetables, legumes, and whole grains
- getting most of your protein from plants rather than animals.
- consuming meals that are minimally processed and as natural as possible and avoiding sugar and sweets
- It also gives one the freedom to occasionally eat meat and other animal products.

Health advantages

Numerous studies have demonstrated that adopting a plant-based diet can lower your chance of contracting chronic illnesses, including type 2 diabetes, while also improving markers of metabolic health. They could also aid with weight loss.

In addition to perhaps aiding in weight loss, flexitarian diets have been demonstrated to lower the risk of type 2 diabetes, enhance metabolic health, blood pressure, and metabolic function.

Other advantages

Reduced meat consumption can help people live more sustainably by lowering greenhouse gas emissions, preventing deforestation, and improving soil quality.

Drawbacks

Transitioning from a more meat-based eating style might make it difficult to maintain plant-based eating habits like vegetarianism and veganism and they may feel restrictive.

Furthermore, while the flexitarian diet is simple to follow because of its flexibility, going overboard with it may have the opposite effect.

Synopsis

Diets based on plants, such as veganism and vegetarianism, may be good for your health. For example, they may lower your chance of developing type 2 diabetes, high blood pressure, and high cholesterol. But for some people, they might also feel limiting.

The flexitarian diet is a less restrictive form of a plant-based diet that permits a small amount of ingestion of meat and other animal products.

4. The MIND diet

To establish an eating pattern that focuses on brain health, the **Mediterranean-DASH Intervention for Neurodegenerative Delay** (MIND) diet combines elements of the DASH and Mediterranean diets.

What it does

The MIND diet, like the flexitarian diet, does not include a rigid meal plan but instead promotes eating 10 certain foods that are good for the brain.

MIND includes eating every week.

- six or more portions of leafy green vegetables daily
- one serving of vegetables that aren't starchy
- five servings or more of nuts

It also promotes the following foods several times per week:

- berries
- beans
- whole grains
- olive oil
- fish

- poultry

Health advantages

According to research, the MIND diet is superior to other plant-rich diets for enhancing cognition and may lower a person's risk of getting Alzheimer's disease.

Additionally, studies indicate that the MIND diet can strengthen older persons' resilience and decrease the progression of cognitive deterioration.

Additionally, it might postpone the start of Parkinson's disease, a movement illness.

The MIND diet and weight loss are topics with limited research. The MIND diet, however, may also assist you in losing weight because it combines two diets that encourage weight reduction.

Encouraging you to limit your consumption of certain foods, it can aid in weight loss in one way or another. These includes

- butter,
- cheese,
- fried foods
- red meat, and
- sweets

The MIND diet and weight loss, however, require more investigation.

Other advantages

The MIND diet has a lot to offer and allows some more flexibility than harsher diets because it combines the best elements of two different diets.

Although you are free to consume outside of the suggested 10 food groups, your results may be better if you adhere to the diet more closely.

Summary

The MIND diet incorporates elements of the DASH and Mediterranean diets and may lower your risk of dementia and Alzheimer's disease.

To determine whether it can aid in weight loss, more study is required.

5. WW (formerly Weight Watchers)

One of the most well-known weight loss programs in the world is WW, formerly known as Weight Watchers.

While there are no food restrictions on the WW plan, participants must stick to their daily point budget to reach their goal weight.

What it does

With the use of a points-based system called WW, various foods and drinks are given values based on their calorie, fat, and fiber levels.

You must adhere to your daily point allotment while you attempt to achieve your ideal weight.

Health advantages

Numerous research supports the idea that the WW program can aid in weight loss.

People who followed the WW diet, for instance, lost 2.6% more weight than those who received normal counseling, according to an analysis of 45 research.

Furthermore, compared to those who adhere to other diets, those who follow WW programs have been demonstrated to be more successful at maintaining weight loss after several years.

Other advantages

Because WW allows for flexibility, it is simple to implement. This makes it possible for folks with dietary restrictions, such as those who have food allergies, to follow the plan.

Downsides

While WW offers flexibility, depending on your membership package and how long you expect to use it, it may be expensive.

According to studies, it may take up to 52 weeks to significantly reduce weight and have clinical advantages.

Additionally, if dieters choose unhealthy foods, their flexibility may be a drawback.

Summary

Weight Watchers, also known as WW, is a points-based weight loss and good eating program.

It is highly versatile and successful for long-term weight loss, according to studies.

6. Intermittent fasting

An eating plan known as intermittent fasting alternates between periods of fasting and eating.

There are many types, such as the 16/8 technique, which calls for consuming no more than 800 calories in any given eight-hour period. The 5:2 approach limits your daily calorie intake to 500–600 calories twice a week.

Intermittent fasting, though generally associated with weight loss, may offer significant advantages for your body and brain.

What it does

Your window for eating is constrained by intermittent fasting, which is an easy approach to cutting calories. If you don't compensate by overeating during permitted eating times, this may result in weight reduction.

Health advantages

Numerous advantages of intermittent fasting include lower inflammation, enhanced brain health, increased insulin sensitivity, and anti-aging effects.

Intermittent fasting may improve heart health and lengthen lifespan, according to studies conducted on both animals and humans.

Additionally, it can aid with weight loss.

Intermittent fasting was found to result in weight loss of between 0.8 and 13% over two weeks to a year in a review of research. This has a much higher proportion than many other approaches.

Other research shows that intermittent fasting can boost metabolism by increasing fat burning while maintaining muscular mass.

Other advantages

Intermittent fasting is regarded as a less complicated eating strategy to follow than other diets that can have several regulations, necessitate frequent excursions to the food store, and be challenging to adhere to.

There are fewer meals that you need to prepare, cook, and clean up after because of the diet's nature.

Downsides

For the majority of healthy persons, intermittent fasting is generally safe.

However, before beginning intermittent fasting, people who are vulnerable to blood sugar decreases should consult a doctor. People in these groups include:

- those who have diabetes,

- are underweight,
- have an eating disorder,
- are pregnant and
- are breast- or bottle-feeding,

Summary

Cycles of intermittent fasting between times when you can eat.

It has been connected to numerous additional health advantages as well as being proven to help with weight loss.

7. The Volumetrics diet

Professor of nutrition at Penn State University Barbara Rolls developed the Volumetrics diet, which is intended to be a long-term lifestyle change rather than a severe eating regimen.

What it does

The eating plan encourages you to load up on nutrient-dense foods that are low in calories and high in water to promote weight loss.

It also restricts items high in calories, such as cookies, candies, nuts, seeds, and oils.

Using a system developed by Rolls, the Volumetrics diet classifies food into four groups depending on its calorie density. These groups include:

- Foods with a very low-calorie density fall under **category one**, such as non-starchy fruits and vegetables, nonfat milk, and broth-based soups.

- Foods in **category two** are low in calories and high in fiber, such as starchy fruits and vegetables, grains, cereal, low-fat meat, beans, and low-fat mixed dishes like chili.

- Foods in **category three** are moderately calorically dense and include things like meat, cheese, pizza, bread, and ice cream.

- High-calorie foods in **category four** include crackers, chips, chocolate sweets, almonds, butter, and oil.

On the volumetric diet, foods from categories one and two make up the majority of the meals, with small amounts of items from categories three and four.

The Volumetrics diet does not fully forbid any meals, and daily activity of at least 30 to 60 minutes is recommended.

Health advantages

The Volumetrics diet promotes nutrient-dense foods that are high in fiber, vitamins, and minerals while being low in calories, which may help you consume more important nutrients and guard against nutritional deficiencies.

Low-calorie-density diets have also been linked in research to better diet quality.

Additionally, it restricts the number of processed foods you consume, lowering your risk of heart disease and some malignancies.

You could lose weight by following the Volumetrics diet.

A meta-analysis of 13 research involving more than 3,000 participants discovered that diets high in low-calorie density foods promoted weight loss. Similar results were reported in an 8-year study including more than 50,000 women, who gained more weight when eating items high in calories.

Downsides

The Volumetrics diet may be beneficial for health and weight loss, but it necessitates an in-depth knowledge of volumetrics, which involves knowing about the calories in foods about portion sizes and nutritional levels.

Some people might find this easier than others.

SUMMARY By encouraging you to fill up on nutrient-dense foods that are low in calories and high in water, The Volumetrics is intended to encourage weight loss.

While it might aid in weight loss, it necessitates a solid grasp of volumetrics and food calorie counts.

8. The Mayo Clinic Diet

The reputable healthcare institution of the same name, the Mayo Clinic, developed the Mayo Clinic Diet.

What it does

The Mayo Clinic Diet focuses on replacing less
healthful behaviors with ones that are more
likely to enhance longevity and weight loss. It is
intended to be a lifestyle adjustment rather than
a quick fix.

The Mayo Clinic Diet uses a pyramid to promote
activity and show the recommended dietary
portions, as opposed to forbidding particular
foods.

The pyramid's foundation is composed of fruits,
vegetables, and physical exercise. The following
layer is composed of carbohydrates, then comes
protein, dairy, fats, and eventually sweets.

There are two phases to the diet. a first,
two-week phase that aims to jump-start your
weight loss by introducing five healthier
behaviors and enticing you to give up five
typical unhealthy ones.

The second stage focuses more on adopting a
long-term lifestyle change and encourages

knowledge of nourishing food selections, portion control, and physical activity.

Health advantages

The Mayo Clinic Diet's advantages for health have not been well studied.

However, the Mayo Clinic advises users to anticipate losing up to 2 pounds during the second phase and roughly 10 pounds during the first two weeks.

The Mayo Clinic Diet may aid in weight loss because it can promote satiety by making you feel more satisfied. It might also lessen your chance of getting type 2 diabetes.

A lower-calorie diet combined with exercise promotes weight loss more effectively than dieting alone, according to studies.

To find out whether the Mayo Clinic Diet is beneficial for helping people lose weight, more research is necessary.

Downsides

The digital version of the program costs money each month to subscribe to, but it comes with meal plans, recipes, a food tracker, virtual group sessions, at-home workouts, and more.

Summary

The Mayo Clinic Diet promotes activity and a diet high in fruits and vegetables by using an easy-to-follow pyramid.

Although the diet's authors advise participants to anticipate losing roughly 10 pounds in the first two weeks, additional research is required to completely comprehend the diet's health advantages.

9. Low carb diets

One of the most well-liked diets for weight loss is the low-carb approach. The Atkins diet, the ketogenic (keto) diet, and the low-carb, high-fat (LCHF) diet are a few examples.

More dramatically than others, some kinds cut carbohydrates. For instance, ultra-low carbohydrate diets like the keto diet cap this macronutrient at less than 10% of total calories, vs 30% or less for other types.

What it does

Diets low in carbohydrates encourage you to eat more protein and fat.

They often contain more protein than low-fat diets, which is crucial since protein can help you lose weight by preserving muscle mass, reducing appetite, and increasing metabolism.

Your body starts turning fatty acids into ketones, which it uses as fuel when you follow very low-carb diets like the ketogenic diet. We refer to this process as ketosis.

Health advantages

According to research, low-carb diets may lessen heart disease risk factors like high blood pressure and cholesterol. They might also lower type 2 diabetics' blood sugar and insulin levels.

Numerous research suggests that low-carb diets may be more effective than traditional low-fat diets for promoting weight loss.

For instance, an analysis of 53 research with 68,128 participants revealed that low-carb diets significantly increased weight loss compared to low-fat diets.

Additionally, low-carb diets seem to be very successful at shedding unhealthy belly fat.

Downsides

A low-carb diet may occasionally cause levels of LDL (bad) cholesterol to increase. Very low carbohydrate diets can also be challenging to stick to and, in some cases, irritate the digestive system (56 Reliable Source).

Very rarely, eating very few carbohydrates may result in ketoacidosis, a serious metabolic disorder that can be fatal if left untreated.

Summary

By limiting your intake of carbohydrates, low-carb diets urge your body to burn more fat for energy.

They have a lot of advantages, including helping you lose weight.

The conclusion

Numerous diets can aid in weight loss and have special health advantages.

The Mediterranean diet, WW (Weight Watchers), the MIND diet, the DASH diet, intermittent fasting, plant-based diets, low-carb diets, the Mayo Clinic Diet, and the Volumetrics diet are a few of the most well-liked eating regimens.

The diet you choose should be based on your lifestyle and dietary choices, even though all of the aforementioned diets have been proven to be successful in helping people lose weight. As a result, you are more likely to maintain it over time.

Additionally, it's always a good idea to discuss your personal health history with your doctor before beginning any new diet. They can assist you in selecting the strategy that will work best for you.

A trained dietician can also assist you in navigating the new guidelines and helping you prepare meals that you want to eat once you've decided to start a new day.

Chapter 5: Healthy Foods For Weight Loss

Consuming meals high in nutrients, such as lean protein and legumes, can improve your general health and assist you in maintaining a healthy weight.

All sizes and types of healthy bodies are possible. Even though weight loss is not a panacea for health and not everyone needs to pursue it, you might want to work toward it if you want to feel the healthiest.

Your diet can influence your health outcomes when combined with regular exercise.

Cutting calories when trying to reduce weight may be tempting, but doing so might be harmful to your health. Studies show that eating less than 1,000 calories per day frequently falls short of giving your body the balanced nourishment it requires and can result in vitamin and mineral shortages linked to major health problems[1].

Furthermore, when you consume much fewer calories than you require, your body starts using its own muscle and organ tissues as fuel. Additionally, your metabolic rate will be slower the less lean tissue mass you have, which is not good for weight loss.

Therefore, focusing on feeding your body better meals is a more successful weight loss technique than controlling your caloric intake. Here are the foods that professionals and scientists agree will promote a healthy and long-lasting weight loss plan.

The Function of Food in Weight Loss

According to Matthew Olesiak, M.D., chief medical director of Bellevue, Washington-based SANESolution, weight regulation is mostly a hormonal reaction to specific foods. "Hormones send signals to the brain that influence our

cravings, hunger, and body weight," he claims.
The impact of various foods on your hunger
hormones is as follows:

Protein makes you feel full fast and for a very
long period. Additionally, it inhibits ghrelin, the
hormone that causes hunger, from being secreted
after meals.

In addition to increasing lean muscle mass and
requiring more energy to process, protein also
speeds up metabolism.

According to Dr. Olesiak, **dietary fiber** slows
down digestion and promotes a gradual rise in
blood glucose levels, which delays the release of
the hormone insulin, which promotes fat storage.

"Various satiety hormones (like ghrelin) are
released as fiber moves through the digestive
system, sending signals to the brain to reduce
hunger and regulate food intake," he claims.

According to certified dietitian Kara Landau, this can cause you to feel fuller for a longer time, which can assist to prevent overeating and lower your overall calorie intake. She continues, "Prebiotic soluble fiber also feeds the good bacteria in your large intestine, which enhances gut health.

Ultra-processed meals have little nutritional value and fiber, which causes them to digest quickly. Consuming them, such as potato chips, candy bars, and toaster pastries, therefore results in a sharp increase in blood glucose levels and a large insulin release," he explains. The majority of those calories go to your fat cells because insulin has to quickly remove glucose from your bloodstream, he says.

"Ideally, you'll use some of these saved calories the following time you need fuel. But if you consume a continuous diet of highly processed foods, you'll always add to your fat reserves rather than remove any of them.

How to Safely and Permanently Lose Weight?

Significant calorie restriction is not required, and it is not recommended either. The healthiest and most long-lasting method of weight loss is to **consume full, unprocessed, high-quality foods.** These foods help you feel fuller longer, speed up your metabolism, and burn fat naturally.

Feit continues, "**Avoid as many processed foods, fried foods, and refined sugars as you can, and be mindful of portion size.**" Using the plate technique, she advises, in which half of your plate is made up of fruits and vegetables, a quarter of lean protein, and a quarter of fiber-rich carbohydrates.

According to Landau, eating a variety of unprocessed, clean meals can also help your gut health. In addition to improving immunity and decreasing inflammation, which will make you feel better physically and mentally and help you stay on track to lose weight, good gut health is also associated with a stronger insulin response (which reduces fat stored around the midsection).

1. Complete eggs

Whole eggs, often despised for their high cholesterol content, have recently become more popular.

These anxieties sprang from misunderstandings that neglected how your body controls cholesterol levels. To keep its baseline levels, your body gets it from your diet or your liver as needed.

While those who already have high levels of LDL (bad) cholesterol should be very careful about how much cholesterol they consume, moderate egg consumption, or 7 to 12 eggs per week, is safe for most people.

Eggs are one of the healthiest meals to eat if you're trying to reach or maintain a healthier weight, even if a larger diet of eggs may increase LDL cholesterol levels in certain people.

Eggs are very nutrient-dense foods. Interestingly, although egg whites provide 4-6 grams of protein each, practically all of its nutrients, including choline and vitamin D, are concentrated in the yolks.

They give you the feeling of being full because they are high in protein and fat.

That's important because it can help you achieve or maintain a healthy weight if you pay attention to your body's internal fullness and hunger cues. To put it another way, developing the practice of just eating when you're hungry and ending when you're full can aid in your weight loss efforts.

In contrast to cereal, milk, and orange juice, eating eggs and buttered toast for breakfast boosted feelings of satiety (fullness) for the following four hours, according to a study including 50 healthy persons with more weight.

An egg-based breakfast that was high or moderate in both protein and fiber was associated with greater feelings of satiety than low-fiber cereal and milk, according to another research of 48 healthy people.

Eating eggs may support your weight loss objectives while also providing you with a wealth of nutritious ingredients since feeling satisfied can help prevent overeating triggered by feeling overly hungry.

2. Leafy vegetables

Kale, spinach, collard greens, Swiss chard, and a few other vegetables are examples of leafy greens.

They are ideal for achieving or maintaining a healthy weight thanks to several characteristics.

For instance, they include minerals and fiber that keep you hydrated and satisfied.

Additionally, leafy greens include thylakoids, plant substances that have been connected to improved appetite control and enhanced fullness in at least two human studies.

The participants in both studies took a 5-gram thylakoid supplement, which is equivalent to around 3.5 ounces (100 grams) of raw spinach. It is important to note, however, that both studies are small.

Those who took the supplement, even only one dose, reported improved hunger control and weight loss.

The effectiveness of thylakoids derived from food sources as a strategy for achieving a healthy weight — as well as their long-term impacts in supplement form — still requires more study in people.

Meanwhile, leafy greens are virtually always an excellent complement to your diet because they contain a variety of fiber and minerals.

You might feel fuller for longer and have fewer cravings for less nourishing foods by increasing your intake of leafy greens. Your longer-term, healthy weight loss objectives can be helped by developing a response to your body's internal indications of hunger and fullness.

You should see a healthcare provider or a qualified dietitian about how many servings of leafy greens you should consume each day if you take drugs, such as blood thinners like warfarin (Coumadin).

Vitamin K, which is abundant in leafy greens and may interfere with your prescription. The key is regular vitamin K intake.

3. Salmon

Salmon and other fatty fish are wonderfully nourishing and filling.

Salmon is a rich source of high-quality protein, beneficial lipids, and several critical elements. This combo keeps you full and can aid in weight loss (18 Trusted Source).

Omega-3 fatty acids, which are abundant in salmon, may help lessen inflammation. Obesity and metabolic disorders are both significantly influenced by inflammation.

Additionally, fish and seafood in general may contain a sizable amount of iodine.

The nutrient is required for healthy thyroid function, which is vital to maintain a healthy metabolism.

However, research indicates that a sizable portion of people do not meet their iodine requirements. You can get adequate iodine by increasing the amount of fatty fish in your diet.

Other fatty fish, such as mackerel, trout, sardines, herring, tuna, and others, are also very good for your health.

4. Vegetables with crucifers

Broccoli, cauliflower, cabbage, and Brussels sprouts are cruciferous vegetables.

They tend to be quite filling and high in fiber, just like other vegetables.

Additionally, these vegetables have a respectable protein content. Even though they are not nearly as high in protein as meat or beans, they are nonetheless high for vegetables.

Cruciferous vegetables are the ideal foods to include in your meals if you want to lose weight because they have a high protein content, fiber content, and low energy density (low calorie content).

They also include nutrients that may reduce your risk of developing cancer and are very healthy. But remember, no amount of cruciferous veggies may take the place of advised cancer screenings or appropriate cancer treatment.

5. A few lean meats and chicken breast

For many, the meat food group is still debatable.

Beyond concerns with ethics and sustainability, it is still unknown whether or how red meat increases the risk of heart disease or diabetes.

There is little proof that eating meat affects health outcomes, according to research.

It's difficult to understand this phrase, and it's frequently taken to mean that eating more meat is a good idea, but it actually only means that there isn't enough data to determine if it has a negative impact on health.

However, consuming a lot of red and processed meat raises your risk of developing cancer, diabetes, heart disease, and dying too soon.

Consuming fruits, vegetables, and whole grains combined with unprocessed meat in moderation (i.e., 2-3 servings per week) may help reduce some of the cancer risks connected with meat consumption.

In terms of nutrition, chicken and red meat both include a lot of protein and iron.

Lean red meat cuts like tenderloin or flank steak that are skinless and packed with protein and iron have less saturated fat than other cuts. To more effectively promote weight control and heart health, choose these the majority of the time.

According to some theories, inflammation, which is linked to chronic illness, is fueled by saturated fat. However, research into this has also so far shown conflicting findings.

The results of your diet can also have an impact
on your health.

When red meat is cooked at high temperatures
for an extended period of time—by smoking or
grilling, for example—fat drippings are
produced. These react with hot cooking surfaces
to produce polycyclic aromatic hydrocarbons
(PAHs), a hazardous byproduct that can lead to
cancer.

Limit your exposure to smoking, clean up spills,
and consume lean meat in moderation to lower
your risk. This implies a weekly limit of a few
3-ounce (85-gram) meals. A serving is around
the size of your hand's palm.

6. Potatoes and other root vegetables

The popularity of lower carb diets may be at
least partially to blame for the apparent decline
in demand for white potatoes.

For what it's worth, potatoes and other root vegetables have a number of benefits that make them excellent sources of nutrients for promoting healthy weight loss.

They include a small amount of practically every nutrient you require and a remarkably wide variety of nutrients.

They are especially rich in potassium, a vitamin that is typically under-consumed. In the control of blood pressure, potassium is crucial.

Boiling white potatoes had the highest rating of any food tested on a scale called the Satiety Index that gauges how full various foods are.

This implies that eating cooked white or sweet potatoes increases the likelihood that you will naturally feel satisfied afterward. Additionally, you'll be giving your body the nutrition it needs.

After boiling, potatoes will produce large amounts of resistant starch, a material that

resembles fiber and has been linked to a number
of health advantages, including weight loss.

Other wonderful options include sweet potatoes,
turnips, and other root vegetables.

7. Tuna

Another filling, high-protein dish is tuna.

Since it is a lean fish, it contains both good fats
and protein, which keeps you feeling full.
Docosahexaenoic acid (DHA), an omega-3 fatty
acid that may be good for your heart, is one of
these beneficial fats.

Eating fish like salmon and tuna can be a
fantastic way to improve your protein intake
while also providing your eyes and brain with
healthy fish fats.

If you want to consume less calories, pick tuna
variants that are canned in water. Oil-packed
tuna contains more calories, fat, and sodium but

might also be more satisfying. Depending on what you need on that particular day.

8. Legumes and beans

Legumes like beans and other legumes can help you lose weight. Lentils, black beans, kidney beans, and various other beans are examples of them.

Those foods frequently have significant levels of protein and fiber, two nutrients that encourage satiety. They frequently include some resistant starch as well.

Because of their high fiber content, beans might make some people feel bloated and gassy. However, careful preparation can lessen these negative effects. Consider purchasing dried beans and soaking them for several hours prior to cooking.

9. Soups

A delightful method to enhance your consumption of whole grains and vegetables that you would not otherwise get enough of is through soup. However, cream-based soups and variants that use processed meats won't offer the same nutritious benefit.

Some people take longer to eat soup than other dishes because of the slurping, sniffing, tasting, cooling, and chewing. You might eat more deliberately if you eat more slowly. Additionally, it might prevent you from overeating.

Reaching and maintaining a healthy weight depend on you feeling full and nourishing your body while paying attention to and acting on your body's hunger and fullness cues.

There are ways to make soup creamier without using heavy cream, which can contribute less beneficial saturated fat, if you like a richer soup.

Consider mixing in avocado, which enhances your soup's fiber content, or cashews. As a

garnish for the soup, you may add slice an
avocado on top.

Soups could help you feel fuller and control your weight because they are naturally watery and hydrate you. Before a meal, try include a clear soup with a vegetable basis to increase feeling of fullness and promote healthy weight loss.

Be aware
When it comes to nutrition, trying to "do it right" may seem alluring, but it might backfire. Consider asking for help if you frequently follow restrictive diets, are always worried about your weight or food, feel guilty about your dietary decisions, or are preoccupied with these issues. These actions could be a sign of an eating disorder or a disordered relationship with food.

10. Cottage cheese

Protein content is often high in dairy products.

Cottage cheese, which is mainly protein, is one of the dairy products with the highest protein content.

You may increase your protein intake, which is crucial for developing and maintaining muscle, by eating cottage cheese. Additionally, it is abundant in calcium and quite filling.

More research is required to determine whether there is a connection between calcium intake and a healthy weight.

Greek yogurt and skyr are two other dairy products with a high protein content.

11. Avocados

Avocados are a distinctive fruit.

The majority of fruits are high in carbohydrates, however, avocados are full of good fats. They have particularly high levels of the monounsaturated oleic acid found in olive oil.

Despite having a high-fat content, avocados are also very satiating due to their high water and fiber content.

Additionally, studies show that their fat content can improve the amount of carotenoid antioxidants your body gets from plants, making them the ideal complement to salads made primarily of veggies. In fact, according to 54Trusted Source, it might boost absorption by 4.6–12.6 times.

They aid in the absorption of other critical fat-soluble vitamins, including vitamins A, D, E, and K. In addition, avocados are a great source of potassium and fiber.

It's important to remember that avocados are high in energy, so if weight loss is your aim, portion control is essential. The more you get used to listening to your body's internal signs for hunger and fullness, the better your intuitive

sense of how much is right for you at that
moment will be.

12. Nuts

In addition to having a high-fat content, nuts also
include fiber, protein, and other plant chemicals
that are good for your heart.

Since they have proportionate amounts of
protein, fiber, and healthy fats, they make great
snacks.

Nut consumption has been linked to better
metabolic health and even weight loss.

Furthermore, research on the general population
has revealed that those who consume nuts tend
to consume more nutrients and maintain a
healthier weight than those who do not.

You should be careful to eat only until you feel
full when consuming this cuisine, as you do with
any high-fat food. So, if your objective is to

reduce weight, be mindful of your portion proportions.

At first, try eating a handful of unsalted nuts. Then, in 15 to 20 minutes, check how you're feeling. Give yourself some time to digest and try half of another handful if you're still hungry.

13. Whole grains

A diet high in whole grains, according to recent studies, can encourage healthy weight loss.

Cereal grains can be nutritious additions to your diet and may be good for your metabolism

That is a result of their high fiber and respectable protein content. A few examples are quinoa, brown rice, and oats.

Oats include a lot of beta-glucans, soluble fibers that may promote metabolic health and increase satiety.

Resistant starch can be found in both brown and white rice, especially if it is cooked and then allowed to cool.

While white rice is undoubtedly OK, brown rice contains extra nutrients, particularly fiber, which may aid in your healthy weight loss efforts.

Refined grains, such as white bread and the majority of commercial baked goods, are acceptable as long as they are consumed in moderation and not as the main component of your diet.

Also keep in mind that some items labeled "whole grain" on the label may be highly processed and, if consumed in excess, may lead to undesirable weight gain.

14. Chili peppers.

Consuming chili peppers can be beneficial while trying to lose weight.

They contain capsaicin, which gives hot peppers like chilies their spicy flavor.

According to certain research, capsaicin can increase your feeling of fullness and speed up the metabolism of fat in your body. These things could help you on your path to healthy weight loss.

The drug is even offered as a supplement and is a typical component of several widely available weight loss products. This is due to studies suggesting that supplements containing capsaicin may speed up metabolism.

However, a review research indicated that compared to people who did not take capsaicin supplements, this impact only resulted in an additional 33 calories burnt each day on average. Especially concerning capsaicin from food sources, more study is required to understand this effect.

Additionally, those who were used to consuming spicy food showed no reaction, showing that a certain amount of tolerance can develop.

15. Fruit

Fruit is healthful, say the majority of health professionals.

People who consume the most fruits and vegetables tend to be healthier than those who don't, according to numerous demographic studies.

The majority of fruits have qualities that make them excellent for aiding in the attainment or maintenance of a healthy weight. Therefore, there's no need to avoid them on your road to health.

Despite having natural sugar, fruits are low in energy density and rich in micronutrients. Additionally, the fiber in them slows down the release of sugar into the bloodstream.

Those who are on an extremely low-carb diet or who have an intolerance may wish to avoid or limit fruit. The majority of fruits can help you achieve a healthy weight goal while also being delightful complements.

16. Grapefruit

Fruits like grapefruit, which are rich in nutrients and fiber, can encourage feelings of fullness.

Eating half of a fresh grapefruit before meals resulted in a weight loss of 3.5 pounds (1.6 kg) in an earlier study from 2006 that followed 91 obese people for 12 weeks.

A metabolic disorder called insulin resistance was also less prevalent in the grapefruit group.

Therefore, consuming half a grapefruit 30 minutes before meals may help you feel fuller and consume fewer calories overall. You might be better off eating a variety of fruits and vegetables at each meal, though, as this is not a sustainable.

If you use certain drugs, such as statins or blood pressure meds, avoid grapefruit and its juice as it can enhance or interfere with their effects.

More studies on humans are still required to fully understand how grapefruit affects weight loss and weight management.

17. Chia seeds

One of the world's most nutrient-dense foods may be chia seeds.

Each ounce (28 grams) has 12 grams of carbohydrates, over 10 of which are fiber.

As a result, chia seeds are a low-carb snack that also happens to include 35% of the world's greatest sources of fiber.

Chia seeds swell and become gel-like in your stomach as a result of their high fiber content.

A mid-morning snack of either 0.33 ounces (7 grams) or 0.5 ounces (14 grams) of chia seeds with yogurt was observed to boost feelings of fullness in one research of 24 individuals.

Additionally, the high omega-3 fatty acid content of chia seeds may help with weight management.

Chia seeds may help you achieve a healthy weight because of their nutritious profile.

18. Whole, full-fat Greek yogurt

Another great dairy product is yogurt.

Given that it contains twice as much protein as conventional yogurt, Greek yogurt is particularly excellent for weight management.

Additionally, some yogurt varieties, such as Greek yogurt, contain probiotic bacteria that can enhance the health of your gut.

To further improve gut health, look for labels that mention "live cultures" or "active cultures." If you don't see these, seek a combination of probiotic strains in the ingredients list, such as S. thermophilus or Bifidus.

Leptin resistance, one of the main hormonal causes of obesity, as well as inflammation may be prevented by having a healthy gut.

Choose yogurt with live, active cultures instead of other varieties, which may have little or no probiotics.

Also, think about selecting full-fat yogurt. Full-fat dairy consumption, but not low-fat dairy, has been linked to a decreased risk of obesity and type 2 diabetes over time, although the evidence for this association is still conflicting.

It's advised to eat flavored or sweetened low-fat yogurt only sometimes and to read the nutrition label if you're trying to avoid those ingredients as they usually have fillers or extra sugars to make up for texture.

19. Lean protein

According to Feit, lean protein sources like chicken, turkey, and grass-fed lean beef help you feel full, reduce cravings, and regulate blood sugar. The same advantages apply to plant-based proteins like legumes, beans, and lentils, and because they are high in fiber, they also encourage satiety.

20. Water

While not a food, water is just as essential for a good weight loss plan. According to Feit, "all of our body processes need water to function—metabolism is one of these processes," so make sure to maintain a healthy hydration level.

The conclusion

Many meals are scrumptious, healthy, and helpful in achieving or maintaining a healthier weight. The majority of them are entire foods, such as fish, lean meat, veggies, fruit, nuts, seeds, and legumes.

Oatmeal and probiotic yogurt are two wonderful examples of minimally processed meals.

Eating these nutritious meals ought to assist in paving the path to a healthy life, along with moderation and regular exercise.

Chapter 6: Smoothies For Weight Loss

A smoothie is a drink that is created by blending several ingredients. A liquid basis, whether fruit juice, milk, yogurt, or ice cream, is a typical component in smoothies. It is possible to add other components, such as fruits, vegetables, non-dairy milk, ice cubes, whey powder, or nutritional supplements.

The components and their amounts in a smoothie will determine how nutritious it is. Large or several portions of fruits and vegetables, which are advised in a balanced diet and meant to replace meals, are frequently included in smoothies. Fruit juice with a lot of sugar, however, might increase calorie consumption and encourage weight gain. You might utilize ingredients like protein powders, sweeteners, or ice cream. Even while smoothies have the same amount of energy as unblended meals, one research revealed that they are less filling.

Types:

1. Green smoothie

A typical green smoothie has 40–50% (approximately half) green vegetables, commonly raw green leafy vegetables like spinach, kale, Swiss chard, collard greens, celery, parsley, or broccoli, with the majority (or all) of the remaining ingredients being fruit. When eaten fresh, the majority of green leafy vegetables have a bitter flavor, however this can be reduced by selecting less bitter veggies (such as baby spinach) or mixing them with sweeter foods.

2. Protein smoothie

Protein powder, water or some other dairy product, fruits, and veggies are all ingredients in a protein smoothie. They are used as a protein supplement for people who want to enhance their protein consumption and may be ingested at any time of the day. When blended alone with milk or water, protein powder might have a gritty flavor. By adding fruit or other sweets, the protein smoothie enhances the flavor of the protein powder.

3. Smoothie with yogurt

A yogurt smoothie is a smoothie that also contains yogurt as a source of protein and to give the beverage a creamy texture. Particularly Greek yogurt is added as a thickening (because of its strained nature) and to benefit from its alleged health advantages.

Smoothies' Health Benefits for Weight Loss

Smoothies provide a variety of other health advantages in addition to accelerating weight reduction.

Here are a few examples:

1. Cleanses the body

Smoothies keep the fiber of fruits and vegetables, unlike liquids. By enhancing antioxidants and improving the activity of enzymes that remove and neutralize free radicals, fiber protects our bodies from poisons. It cleanses your liver and is essential in avoiding the buildup of fat.

According to research, using fibrous fruits and vegetables in your smoothies, such as berries, bananas, pears, beets, leafy greens, etc., helps to remove dangerous waste that has collected between tissues and purifies your blood.

2. Increases immunity

Fresh fruits and vegetables, nuts, and seeds are the main components of a smoothie. These substances are abundant in numerous phytonutrients and minerals that bolster the immune system and edify the body.

Our bodies are shielded from all infections and diseases by an effective immune system. If you get sick, having a stronger immune system will speed up and improve your recovery time.

Additionally, it aids in reducing the consequences of some illnesses, particularly those that are resistant to antibiotics.

3. Boosts Digestion

Fiber is well recognized for making digestion easier and providing the stool more volume, which helps to quickly relieve constipation and other associated problems. You might be surprised to learn that smoothies are easier on the digestive system than raw fruits or veggies.

4. Maintains Hydration

Dehydration occurs when the body has less water than is necessary, which increases your risk of contracting a number of illnesses.

Smoothies replace the water your body loses since they are a blend of different fruits. Smoothies satisfy your dietary requirements while providing you with twice as much hydration as ordinary water.

5. Improves the health of the skin and hair

Smoothies may strengthen your hair and give you better skin. They are an incredible source of vitamins, minerals, antioxidants, and fiber, all of which naturally increase appearance.

These phytonutrient deficiencies have a variety of effects on our skin and hair. Smoothies made from various fruits and vegetables can help battle a variety of skin-related problems, from acne to aging symptoms, when consumed on a regular basis.

Fruits high in antioxidants encourage the creation of collagen and combat free radicals that harm the skin. Additionally, it might lessen hair loss and improve the appearance of hair.

A. Green Smoothies

How come green smoothies?

The fact that green smoothies are so simple to create is one of its best qualities. To get started, all you need is a blender and some fresh or frozen ingredients. Green smoothies are another excellent method to get more greens in your diet. Green smoothies are a terrific method to receive the nutrients your body needs without having to consume leafy greens if you're not a huge fan of doing so.

Do Green Smoothies Aid in Weight Loss?

The ability to aid in weight loss is yet another fantastic benefit of green smoothies. Green smoothies are a great source of fiber and minerals that can help you feel full and content all day. They are an excellent option if you're attempting to reduce weight because they are minimal in calories. Green smoothies can also speed up your metabolism and aid in weight loss.

It's crucial to remember that simply adding a green smoothie to an unhealthy diet won't help you lose weight but including them in a healthy diet and way of life might - especially if you use them to substitute high-calorie or high-fat meals.

How Do You Make a Green Smoothie for Weight Loss?

After going over some of the advantages of green smoothies, let's talk about how to make one. This is a general suggestion for experimenting and making your own delectable, healthy smoothies; it is not a recipe per se.

1. The Foundation

You can use any liquid you like—water, green tea, almond or coconut milk, etc.—as this. To aid in weight loss, aim for a low-calorie, low-fat base, unless you're following the keto diet or any comparable plan, in which case you should focus more on carbohydrates than calories or fat.

Because it has very few calories and contains catechins, a class of antioxidants that have been shown to speed up metabolism and encourage fat loss, green tea is a fantastic option.

Coconut water, which has few calories and includes electrolytes that can help you keep hydrated, is another excellent option.

Use skim milk or low-calorie plant-based milk (I prefer Simply Almond unsweetened almond milk) if you prefer a creamier smoothie.

2. Add Green Leafy Vegetables.

The majority of your nutrition will come from here. Dark leafy greens are a great source of antioxidants, vitamins, and minerals. They're a fantastic source of fiber, which can help you feel full and content all day long.

Fresh spinach, kale, and Swiss chard are some of my preferred leafy greens to incorporate into green smoothies. Try experimenting with various greens like arugula, collard greens, and dandelion greens (excellent for detox smoothies).

When making green smoothies for the first time, start with a small number of greens and gradually increase it over time. In addition, since spinach blends best in smoothies, I advise beginning with one as your first green. Then you

can gradually progress to a kale smoothie or
another type of green smoothie.

3. Add Some Good Fats.

Any diet should include healthy fats, but losing
weight is a situation where they're even more
crucial. By helping you feel full and content
throughout the day, healthy fats can help you
avoid overeating or unhealthy snacking.

Avocado, coconut oil, nut butter like almond or
peanut butter, and chia seeds are excellent
options for healthy fats. If you want to give your
smoothie an extra protein boost, you can also
add a scoop of protein powder or some Greek
yogurt.

Fruit and Sweets To The Mix

Fruits are a terrific way to give your green
smoothies sweetness and taste. They are a good

source of vitamins, minerals, antioxidants, and dietary fiber.

The majority of your fruit should be lower sugar options like berries, apples, and citrus fruits, but you can also include a small amount of pineapple, mango, and banana. In my smoothies, frozen bananas are my absolute favorite.

Although frozen fruit (such as frozen mango, frozen banana, etc.) will give your smoothie the best texture, you can also use fresh fruit.

You can also add a small amount of honey, maple syrup, monk fruit, stevia, or agave syrup to your smoothie if you think it needs more sweetness. Two or three pitted dates work well as a natural sweetener.

Finally, if desired, add some ice and process the mixture until it is smooth. Ice shouldn't be required if frozen fruit is used.

That's all, then! You now have a healthy, tasty green smoothie that can aid in weight loss.

Green Smoothies for Weight Loss: Benefits

Because **they are loaded with nutrients and fiber** that can keep you full all day, green smoothies are a great way to lose weight. They are a fantastic option for people wanting to reduce weight because **they are also low in calories.**

Green smoothies also have the advantage of being a **wonderful source of antioxidants**, which can assist safeguard your body from illness and advance general wellness.

Last but not least, a terrific way to get your recommended **daily intake of greens** is through green smoothies! The nutrients included in dark leafy greens, including folate and vitamin K, as well as minerals and antioxidants, are vital for maintaining good health. Green smoothies are a great option if you're seeking a delicious and wholesome approach to reducing weight.

How to Include Green Smoothies in Your Diet and Way of Life

Green smoothies are a fantastic option if you're trying to lose weight. Finding ways to include them in your everyday activities is crucial if you want to make them a part of your diet and lifestyle. Here are a few pieces of advice:

To be able to create a green smoothie whenever the urge strikes, make sure you have all the necessary components on hand.

Green smoothies can be prepared in bulk and kept in the refrigerator for an easy and nutritious snack or dinner if you're pressed for time. (However, for optimal benefits, consume within 24 hours or freeze)

As part of a healthy diet and way of life, consume green smoothies. Include additional nutrient-dense foods like whole grains, lean protein, and fruits and vegetables.

Try out new flavor combinations and be inventive with your green smoothies. There are countless options available!

Allow yourself some time to get used to the flavor of green smoothies by being patient. Start with a little amount of greens and gradually add more if you're not used to drinking them.

Finally, but certainly, not least, remember to enjoy your green smoothies! Find what works for you and stick with it because this is a lifestyle change rather than a quick-fix diet.

Advice on Maintaining Your Weight Loss Goals

Green smoothies might be a terrific addition to your diet if you're trying to lose weight. However, it's crucial to position yourself for success by making a few small lifestyle changes to ensure your success. Here are a few bits of advice:

1. Ensure that you are getting adequate water. This is particularly crucial if you want to lose weight. Try to drink 8 to 10 glasses of water each day.

2.Daily breakfast is a must. Your metabolism will be boosted, and you won't feel the need to snack later in the day. A green smoothie with protein and good fat is a great breakfast choice, as you can see!

3. Make time to work out. Exercise will help you raise your metabolism and burn more calories, even if it's simply a 30-minute walk.

4. Steer clear of processed foods, sugary beverages, and excessive alcohol

consumption. These things can all hinder your attempts to lose weight.

5. Maintain a balanced diet. Consuming a lot of fruits, vegetables, whole grains, lean protein, and healthy fats is necessary to achieve this.

6. Maintain a food diary. This will enable you to monitor your progress and, if necessary, alter your diet to achieve the desired outcomes.

7. Find a network of support. Having people to support and inspire you, whether they be family, friends, or members of an online community, can make all the difference in your success.

A fantastic strategy to get healthy and accomplish your goals is to include green smoothies in your weight loss regimen. You'll achieve achievement quickly if you heed this advice!

Use this simple recipe to learn how to create green smoothies for weight loss.

Equipment:
measuring tools
blender

Ingredients:
1 serving of new baby spinach
1 kale cup
1 medium banana, frozen
1/4 cup of chunks of frozen mango
Juice from one orange
1 cup of green tea, steeped
10 grams of chia seeds
2 dates (pitted)

Instructions:
Blender with all components added.
Blend until smooth at a high speed.
Enjoy!

B. High-Protein Smoothies

A protein smoothie will keep your body satisfied until lunch and is simple to digest. Not to mention that it tastes fantastic! They are the ideal answer for a fast and simple breakfast that is packed with nutrients and whose flavor never gets old.

Your body wants to break its extended fast in the greatest way possible after eight hours of (hopefully) sound sleep. Smoothies are delicious, easy to digest, and packed with the nutrients the body needs to start the day. This protein smoothie is the ideal morning option if you want something quick and tasty. It can be the ideal approach to fill you up without using a lot of dishes like other breakfast recipes, taking only 10 minutes to prepare.

Best Fruits For Fruit Smoothies With High Protein

Any fruit will work with protein fruit smoothie recipes, which is fantastic. Make your next smoothie with one of these fruits:

- Bananas

- Mangoes

- Strawberries

- Blueberries

- Raspberries

- Pineapple

- Melon

Vegetables and other non-"fruits" provide smoothies a nutritious boost as well. Take spinach, avocado, kale, and cucumber as examples.

Making The Best High Protein Fruit Smoothies: Some Tips

Therefore, the greatest benefit of smoothies is **their high nutritional value and simplicity of preparation. They are scrumptious, packed with fiber, and a fantastic way to speed up weight loss.** Follow these guidelines to create the best high-protein fruit smoothies ever:

• Use unsweetened almond milk (or your preferred milk) as your liquid because it has a good consistency, is low in calories, and is high in vitamins and minerals.

• It usually works best to add your ingredients to your blender in this order: liquid, no frozen fruits or vegetables, greens, if any, frozen fruits and vegetables, and protein powder.

• Add lemon juice if your smoothie seems to be excessively sweet.

• Add pineapple, orange, or banana if the flavor is too bitter.

• Smoothies taste fantastic when natural sweeteners like honey and pure maple syrup are used.

• Avocado can add creaminess and a ton of vitamins to a smoothie.

• The shake is sweeter when the banana is riper.

Best Protein Powder For Fruit Smoothies With High Protein

1. Pea protein: Protein from pulverized yellow split peas is isolated to create pea protein. It is low in methionine but has all the important amino acids. But you can compensate by eating things like eggs, beef, poultry, brown rice, and more. Pea protein is high in iron, however, for optimal results, it should be combined with citrus powders. It has been demonstrated to aid people who train to grow muscle mass and to help them feel fuller.

2. Whey protein: This protein is supposed to aid in weight loss, muscular growth, and strength improvement. Protein known as whey is taken out of milk's whey. As soon as the cheese is formed, it separates from milk. Smoothies frequently include flavored whey as a nice nutritional boost. We know that whey digests fast.

3. Egg proteins: Egg whites, not egg yolks, are typically used to make egg proteins. Eggs are second only to whey in terms of the amount of leucine, an amino acid that is thought to improve muscle strength. It normally has a good grade and is easily digested in protein powders.

4. Casein protein: Like whey, casein protein is a component of milk. It is believed that those who engage in resistance exercise and consume it will have a higher body composition. It allows for additional amino acid exposure to the muscles because it digests and absorbs more slowly than whey protein.

Ways To Add Protein Without Protein Powder

Looking for a non-powder way to add protein to your smoothie? You may solve that easily by adding one of these delectable ingredients:

- Unflavored Greek yogurt

- Cheese cottage

- No-sugar kefir

- Sugar-free soy milk

- Nut butter like almond or peanut butter

- Flax seeds

- Chia seeds

- Eggs whites

- Oatmeal

Recipe for Protein Smoothies

The liquid should always be added first when preparing this high-protein smoothie. Add your liquid first, whether it's non-dairy milk or a fruit drink like orange juice. This will prevent the protein powder from clumping and adhering to the side. Granola can be sprinkled over top to further resemble an acai bowl. It has the most incredible flavor!

1. **Add Milk**: Fill a powerful blender with almond milk.

2. **Add more ingredients**: Banana, blueberries, spinach, protein powder, and then almond butter.

3. Blend on high until the mixture is smooth and creamy. If necessary, add more almond milk to the mixture to aid in blending. To achieve the correct consistency, mix with more ice and almond milk.

How to Keep Smoothies Fresh

Recipes for protein fruit smoothies can be prepared the night before and kept in the refrigerator for the following day. It is better to include the banana, if it is in the recipe, the morning you want to consume it. If not, your smoothie will be an unappealing shade of brown and won't appear as fresh. However, the flavor and nutritional value will remain the same.

Put your smoothie in a glass container if you're using whey or casein protein powder. This is because the plastic, which contains the mix, is absorbent and can start to smell weird if left sitting.

After blending a protein fruit smoothie recipe for premixing, put it in an airtight glass container. Although it will stay fresh for up to 24 hours, for the best flavor, add some frozen fruit to the mixture and reblend it before drinking.

C. Greek Yoghurt Smoothies

Greek yogurt smoothies are beneficial for both weight loss and supplying your body with essential vitamins and nutrients.
Other healthful elements in the smoothie include blueberries.

One of the finest methods to give creaminess and nutrition to your smoothie is by using Greek yogurt.

It contributes to the balance of other types of smoothies, adding depth and richness to green smoothies as well as balancing off the sweetness of fruit smoothies.

Yogurt is a good source of calcium and high-quality protein. Additionally, plain Greek yogurt has gut-friendly bacteria, which are well-known to be very healthy for us. Smoothies made with plain yogurt, rather than flavor-infused varieties, can aid in weight loss.Unfortunately, flavored yogurt has a lot of added sugar and other processed ingredients to give it flavor and color.

Differences of Greek Yogurt From Normal Yogurt

This sort of yogurt differs from conventional yogurt in the following ways thanks to the Greek process:

- **Taste and Texture**: Greek yogurt has a thicker consistency than conventional yogurt, which makes it a perfect thickening for smoothies and a terrific alternative to sour cream and crème fraiche. If you've never had it, give it a try and see how you like it because the flavor is tangier.

- **Carbs**: Greek yogurt has around half as many as regular yogurt does in terms of carbohydrates.Pick the yogurts with the fewest added sugars for the lowest carb count.

- **Protein**: Greek yogurt has about twice as much protein as normal yogurt.This makes it perfect for smoothies after a workout and helps you feel satiated for longer if you're trying to lose weight.

- **Sodium**: Greek yogurt has around half the amount of sodium in it compared to normal yogurt.

- **Fat**: Greek yogurt typically has nearly three times as much saturated fat as normal yogurt. I always go for a low-fat or non-fat option because of this.

Greek yogurt can be found in a variety of flavors, milk fat concentrations, and plain or flavored varieties.

What advantages does Greek yogurt have for your health?

Here are some of the most recent discoveries regarding yogurt's health advantages:

1. Higher protein

However, protein does more than just make yogurt creamier and thicker.

With more protein and amino acids in your diet thanks to yogurt, you'll feel fuller and less hungry. It's also great as a smoothie before or after exercise.

2. Probiotics

Greek yogurt is a wonderful source of conjugated linoleic acid, which some studies have shown to have a preventive impact against breast cancer. It is also a rich source of probiotics for maintaining good gut health.

3. Long-term prevention of illness

Additionally, it could contribute to a lower risk of developing metabolic syndrome, lower the risk of depression, and even improve skin.

Greek yogurt is a fantastic method to thicken smoothies without adding extra sugar or carbohydrates, even without all of that.

The advantages of Greek yogurt are included in these simple smoothie recipes with yogurt, which also offer a delectable meal replacement option at any time of the day.

Recipes for Smoothies Using Greek Yogurt

1. Banana Strawberry Yogurt Smoothie

This is a fantastic protein smoothie with Greek yogurt that you can prepare for breakfast or to boost your protein intake and develop muscle after a challenging workout.

1 smoothie is served.

Ingredients

- 1/2 cup Greek yogurt, plain
- Strawberries, 1 cup
- 12 bananas (you can omit the ice and use frozen)
- 1-tablespoon almond butter
- Vanilla extract, 1/2 tsp, and
- Water, 1/2 cup

Instructions

Blend each ingredient separately until it is smooth and creamy.

2. Yogurt-topped Blueberry Smoothie

This wholesome morning energy boost includes spinach and blueberries in a fresh smoothie.

1 smoothie is served.

Ingredients

- 3 tablespoons of plain Greek yogurt
- 1/2 ripe banana
- Frozen blueberries, 1/3 cup
- 1/2 cup spinach leaves
- 1/4 cup almond milk without sugar
- 1 teaspoon (optional) protein powder

Instructions

Blend each ingredient separately until it is smooth and creamy.

3. Orange Vanilla Smoothie, third

This wonderful, healthy, grown-up smoothie version of the traditional orange creamsicle blends all the pleasures of childhood in one creamy, delightful treat.

1 smoothie is served.

Ingredients

- 1 cup vanilla Greek yogurt
- 1 frozen banana (for even easier use, peel and cut the banana before freezing).
- 1–2 teaspoons vanilla extract
- 1 large orange, peeled and sliced.
- 2 teaspoons orange zest, as required

Instructions

Blend each ingredient until it is smooth, creamy, and thick. It is advised to use a high-performance blender if you are using a frozen banana.

4. Smoothie with Greek yogurt and banana

This creamy smoothie has a straightforward composition and a robust vanilla taste.

1 smoothie is served.

Ingredients:

- Plain, non-fat Greek yogurt, 6 ounces
- Vanilla extract, two drops
- 1 banana, frozen if desired.
- Spinach, 1 cup
- Water, 1/2 cup

Instructions

Blend all the ingredients in a blender until the frozen components are completely incorporated.

5. Greek yogurt with Muscle-Friendly Protein Smoothie

This fruity smoothie has 65 grams of protein and will keep you satisfied. You can experiment with various protein powder flavors. I discovered that vanilla or cookies and cream work well.

1 smoothie is served.

Ingredients

- 1/2 cup plain Greek yogurt
- 1 cored and peeled apple
- 1 serving of protein powder
- 1 mango cup
- 50% of a pineapple
- one cup of water
- 1.5 cups ice

Instructions

The ingredients should be thoroughly blended.

Chapter 7: Healthy Workout Plan For Weight Loss

Numerous forms of exercise can help you lose weight by increasing the number of calories you burn. Depending on your age, nutrition, and beginning weight, you can lose different amounts of weight.

About half of all American adults, according to estimates, make an effort to lose weight each year.

Exercise is one of the most popular methods used by people seeking to lose extra weight, next to diets. It burns calories, which is important for weight loss.

Exercise not only helps you lose weight but also improves your mood, strengthens your bones, and lowers your risk of developing numerous chronic conditions.

The top 8 exercises for losing weight are shown below.

1. Strolling

One of the finest activities for losing weight is walking and for good reason.

It's a practical and simple approach for new exercisers to get started without feeling overwhelmed or having to buy equipment. Additionally, because it is a lower-impact exercise, your joints are not overworked.

A 155-pound (70-kg) person walks at a modest 4 mph (6.4 km/h) for 30 minutes to burn about 175 calories, according to Harvard Health (5).

Walking for 50 to 70 minutes, three times per week, decreased body fat and waist circumference by an average of 1.5% and 1.1

inches (2.8 cm), respectively, in a 12-week trial of 20 obese women.

You may easily incorporate walking into your regular schedule. Try walking during your lunch break, using the stairs at work, or taking extra walks with your dog to increase the number of steps you take each day.

Aim to go for a 30-minute walk three to four times a week to get started. As you get fitter, you can gradually increase the length or frequency of your walks.

Summary

For beginners, walking is an excellent kind of exercise. It doesn't require any equipment, you can do it practically anywhere, and it only slightly strains your joints. Make an effort to take more walks as part of your daily activities.

2. Running or jogging

Running and jogging are excellent exercises for weight loss.

A jogging pace is often between 4-6 mph (6.4-9.7 km/h), whereas a running pace is quicker than 6 mph (9.7 km/h), despite the similarities in appearance.

A 155-pound (70-kg) person is thought to burn about 288 calories per 30 minutes of jogging at a rate of 5 mph (8 km/h) or 360 calories per 30 minutes of running at a pace of 6 mph (9.7 km/h) according to Harvard Health.

Additionally, research has shown that running and jogging can aid in the burning of visceral fat, also referred to as belly fat. Your internal organs are encircled by this sort of fat, which has been linked to numerous chronic illnesses like diabetes and heart disease.

Running and jogging are both excellent activities that you can do anywhere and that you can easily fit into your weekly regimen. Aim to jog for 20 to 30 minutes, three to four times a week, to start.

Try running on softer terrain like grass if you feel that jogging or running outside is difficult on your joints. Additionally, a lot of treadmills come with built-in cushioning, which might be less stressful on your joints.

Summary

Running and jogging are effective weight-loss exercises that fit easily into a schedule. Additionally, they can lessen visceral fat, which has been linked to diabetes, heart disease, and other chronic illnesses.

3. Biking

Cycling is a well-liked workout that boosts fitness and can aid in weight loss.

Cycling is typically an outdoor exercise, although stationary bikes are common in gyms and fitness facilities, allowing you to pedal indoors.

A 155-pound (70 kg) person is thought to burn about 252 calories per 30 minutes of moderately paced stationary cycling or 288 calories per 30 minutes of moderately paced bicycle riding at a speed of 12–13.9 mph (19–22.4 km/h) according to Harvard Health.

Cycling is excellent for losing weight, but research has also shown that regular cyclists have greater general fitness, increased insulin sensitivity, and a decreased risk of heart disease, cancer, and death than non-cyclists.

All fitness levels, from novices to athletes, can benefit from cycling. Additionally, since it doesn't involve any weight-bearing and has a low impact, your joints won't be put under a lot of strain.

Summary

People of all fitness levels should consider cycling. Studies show that frequent cycling lowers the chance of developing several chronic diseases and improves insulin sensitivity.

4. Bodybuilding

People who want to lose weight frequently choose to lift weights.

A 155-pound (70-kg) person exercises for 30 minutes while burning about 108 calories.

Additionally, weight training can increase your resting metabolic rate (RMR), which is the number of calories your body burns while at rest.

One 6-month study found that performing strength-based workouts for just 11 minutes, three times per week, led to an average 7.4% improvement in metabolic rate. According to this study, that improvement amounted to an increase in daily calorie expenditure of 125

Another study discovered that men's metabolic rates increased by 9% after 24 weeks of weight training, or an additional 140 calories per day. Women's metabolic rates rose by over 4%, or 50 extra calories each day.

Additionally, studies have shown that, in contrast to aerobic exercise, your body continues to burn calories for many hours after a weight-training session.

Summary

By burning calories both during and after an exercise, weight training can assist in weight loss. Additionally, it promotes muscle growth, which may increase your resting metabolic rate.

5. Alternating exercises

High-intensity interval training (HIIT), also referred to as interval training, is a general term for brief bursts of intensive exercise that are followed by rest periods.

A HIIT workout typically lasts 10 to 30 minutes and can burn a lot of calories.

HIIT burns 25–30% more calories per minute than other forms of exercise, such as weight training, cycling, and treadmill jogging, according to a study of 9 active males.

This means that HIIT can enable you to exercise less and burn more calories.

Additionally, a large number of studies have demonstrated that HIIT is particularly effective at reducing belly fat, which is linked to several chronic diseases.

Adding HIIT to your exercise program is simple. Simply decide on an activity, such as biking, running, or jumping, as well as your exercise and rest periods.

On a bike, for instance, pedal as hard as you can for 30 seconds, then slowly for one to two minutes. For ten to thirty minutes, repeat this technique.

Summary

You can use interval training, a powerful weight loss technique, with a variety of activities. You can burn more calories in less time by using interval training in a routine.

6. Swimming

A wonderful approach to shedding pounds and toning up is through swimming.

A 155-pound (70-kg) person swimming for 30 minutes is thought to burn around 216 calories by Harvard Health.

It seems that the way you swim affects how many calories you burn. According to research done on competitive swimmers, the breaststroke burns the most calories, followed by the butterfly, backstroke, and freestyle.

Swimming for 60 minutes three times a week for 12 weeks dramatically reduced body fat, increased flexibility, and decreased numerous heart disease risk factors, including high total cholesterol and blood triglycerides in a study of 24 middle-aged women.

Swimming has the added benefit of being low-impact, which is better for your joints. This makes it a fantastic solution for those who experience joint pain or injuries.

Summary

A fantastic low-impact workout for those trying to lose weight is swimming.

7. Yoga

Yoga is a well-liked form of exercise and stress relief.

Although it's not typically thought of as a weight loss exercise, it does burn a decent amount of calories and has many other advantages that can help with weight loss.

A 155-pound (70-kg) person is thought to burn about 144 calories during a 30-minute yoga session, according to Harvard Health (5).

In a 12-week study of 60 obese women, it was shown that those who practiced yoga twice a week for 90 minutes saw bigger decreases in waist circumference than those in the control group — by an average of 1.5 inches (3.8 cm).

The yoga group also noticed changes in their physical and mental health.

In addition to helping you lose weight, research has shown that yoga can help you learn mindfulness and lower your stress.

Yoga classes are typically offered at gyms, but you may do yoga anywhere. This includes doing it from the convenience of your house because there are many instructional videos online.

Summary

Yoga is a fantastic activity for losing weight that you can do practically anyplace.

8. Pilates

Pilates is a wonderful, user-friendly exercise that could aid with weight loss.

In a 30-minute beginner's Pilates session or a 30-minute advanced Pilates class, a person weighing about 140 pounds (64 kg) would burn 108 calories or 168 calories, respectively, according to a study funded by the American Council on Exercise.

Pilates may not burn as many calories as cardiovascular activities like running, but because it's often fun, it's simpler to maintain over time.

When compared to a control group who did no exercise during the same 8-week period, performing Pilates exercises for 90 minutes three times per week significantly reduced waist, stomach, and hip circumference.

Pilates may help you lose weight while also reducing lower back pain and enhancing your general fitness level, strength, balance, and flexibility.

If Pilates sounds interesting to you, consider adding it to your weekly schedule. Pilates can be practiced either at home or in one of the many gyms that provide the program.

Combine Pilates with a healthy diet or other forms of exercise, like weightlifting or cardio, to accelerate weight loss even more.

Summary

Pilates is a wonderful, beginner-friendly activity that can help you get in shape while also assisting with weight loss.

How much weight loss can you anticipate?

Numerous variables affect how much weight you can expect to lose through exercise.

These consist of:

Weight at birth: People who weigh more at birth often have greater basal metabolic rates. This represents the number of calories your body expends while carrying out essential life-supporting procedures. You will burn more calories while active and at rest if your BMR is higher.

Age: Your BMR decreases as you become older since you tend to have less muscle mass and more fat mass. Losing weight may be more challenging if your BMR is lower.

Gender: Women often have a higher ratio of fat to muscle than males, which may have an impact on their BMR. Men typically shed weight more quickly than women do, despite having identical calorie intake.

Diet: When you burn more calories than you take in, you lose weight. So, to lose weight, you must have a calorie deficit.

Sleep: According to studies, getting too little sleep might make it harder to lose weight and can even make you crave more high-calorie foods.

Medical issues: People who suffer from illnesses like depression and hypothyroidism might lose weight more slowly.

Genetic studies have revealed a genetic component to weight loss, which may influence some obese individuals.

Though the majority of people desire rapid weight loss, experts frequently advise losing 1-2 pounds (0.5-1.36 kg), or roughly 1% of your body weight, each week.

Fast weight loss might have detrimental effects on one's health. Dehydration, exhaustion, starvation, migraines, irritability, constipation, hair loss, and irregular periods are just a few of the symptoms it can cause.

Furthermore, those who lose weight too quickly are more likely to gain it back.

It's crucial to remember that losing weight is not a linear process, and it's typical to see greater weight reduction when you first begin.

Summary

How much weight you might expect to lose through exercise depends on a variety of things. The majority of professionals advise dropping 1-3 pounds weekly.

The conclusion

Numerous exercises can aid in weight loss.

Walking, jogging, running, cycling, swimming, weight training, interval training, yoga, and Pilates are all excellent options for burning calories.

Nevertheless, numerous additional exercises can support your efforts to lose weight.

The most crucial thing is to pick an activity you enjoy. This increases the likelihood that you'll continue with it over the long run and see results.

Chapter 8: The Link Between Obesity, Overweight And Sciatica

What is Sciatica?

The sciatic nerves, which go from your spine to the muscles in your leg and foot, are afflicted by the painful ailment known as sciatica. These nerves travel directly from your spinal cord through your legs, buttocks, and feet. Your body has a sciatic nerve on each side.

Due to the position of those nerves, sciatic pain affects a large portion of your back and lower body, rendering many disabled. An irritated sciatic nerve can cause agonizing pain that travels from your back to the bottom of your foot.

You experience a variety of pains on one side of your body when your sciatic nerve is irritated. Injuries can:

- Follow the sciatic nerve.

- Be abrupt, cutting, or firing

- Linger

- Present as tingling and numbness in the legs or feet

- Additionally, if you spend a lot of time sitting, are generally sedentary, or move your body incorrectly or suddenly, your sciatica may get worse.

Sciatica danger signs

Your sciatic nerve might experience pressure for a variety of causes, which can result in sciatica. Sciatica can be caused by a herniated disc, a bone spur, or another ailment that is brought on by engaging in certain physical activities, getting hurt, or simply getting older, but it can also be brought on by perfectly manageable lifestyle choices.

For many patients, sciatic nerve discomfort is exacerbated by factors like weight. Being fat or even merely overweight puts unnecessary pressure on your spine, which can cause sciatica or make it worse. It also takes longer to recover from sciatica if you weigh more than is healthy.

The risks of leaving sciatica untreated

It's impossible to ignore sciatica, and there comes a time when you may start to exhibit symptoms that are pretty serious and require medical attention. If sciatica is not adequately treated or quickly gets worse, you might experience:

- noticeable leg weakness

- impacted bowel or bladder movements

- irreversible nerve damage

- extreme pain

Although it is ideal for sciatica to not get to this degree, there are treatments available for all sciatica severity levels.

Using a comprehensive strategy to treat sciatica

Based on the cause of sciatica, this method frequently recommends a combination of therapies, some of which may include osteopathic manipulation, anti-inflammatory injections, and hot-and-cold compress therapy.

However, if your sciatica is brought on by weight, you can give priority to sensible lifestyle adjustments that will help you lose weight. To aid in weight loss, this may entail nutritional advice, vitamins, and detoxification therapy. You may also want to incorporate physical therapy or low-impact exercise into your routine.

Don't endure unnecessary pain from sciatica.

www.ingramcontent.com/pod-product-compliance
Lightning Source LLC
Chambersburg PA
CBHW061345250726
48657CB00004B/1331